THE MARIA MONTESSORI CENTER, INC.
32450 W. 13 MILE ROAD
FARMINGTON HILLS, MI 48018

Touch and Feeling is about a sense which protects our bodies by letting us know when we are hot or cold or feeling pain. The book explains how the sense of touch works through the skin, nervous system and brain; and the importance of touch to us and to other animals. Simple experiments for further exploration of touch and feeling are also included.

First published in Great Britain in 1985
by Macdonald & Co. (Publishers) Ltd
London & Sydney

A BPCC plc company

Adapted and published in the
United States in 1986 by
Silver Burdett Company,
Morristown, New Jersey

LIBRARY OF CONGRESS CATALOGING IN PUBLICATION DATA

Royston, Robert.
Touch and feeling.

Includes index.
Summary: Explains how the sense of touch works through the skin, nervous system, and brain to register pressure, temperature, texture, and pain. Includes simple experiments for further exploration of touch and feeling.
1. Touch—Juvenile literature. 2. Senses and sensation—Juvenile literature. [1. Touch] I. Title.
QP451.R68 1986 612'.88 85-27834
ISBN 0-382-09176-0

TOUCH AND FEELING

Robert Royston

Silver Burdett Company
Morristown, New Jersey

How to use this book

First, look at the contents page opposite. Read the chapter list to see if it includes the subject you want. The list tells you what each page is about. You can then find the page with the information you need.

If you want to know about one particular thing, look it up in the index on page 31. For example, if you want to know about the cortex, the index tells you that there is something about it on pages 12, 13 and 30. The index also lists the pictures in the book.

When you read this book, you will find some unusual words. The glossary on page 30 explains what they mean.

Series Editor
Margaret Conroy

Book Editor
Margaret Conroy

Series Design
Robert Mathias/Anne Isseyegh

Book Design
Jane Robison

Production
Susan Mead

Picture Research
Caroline Mitchell

Factual Adviser
Dr Geoff Watts

Reading Consultant
Amy Gibbs
Inner London Education Authority
Centre for Language in Primary Education

Teacher Panel
Roger Smith
Ann Merriman

Illustrations
David Eaton Front cover
Mark Lewis Pages 10-15
Michael Robinson Page 9 bottom
Michael Whittlesea Pages 6-9, 16-17, 20-21, 26-27

Photographs
Aldus Archive: cover (except TR)
Arctic Camera: 25
Camerapix Hutchison Library: 29
Institute of Dermatology: 17
Rex Features: 24
RNIB: cover TR
John Watney: 18
ZEFA: 19, 22, 23L & R, 28

CONTENTS

FEELING

What touch tells us

This book is about touch. Touch is one of the five senses, together with sight, hearing, smell and taste.

You use your sense of touch when you reach out your hand and feel an object. If you touch a rose petal it feels soft and silky, if you touch a saw with jagged teeth it feels sharp and dangerous.

But touch tells you other things, too. It makes you feel your muscles stretching when you run. You feel a dizzy shock of cold when you jump into a swimming pool. If you fall off your bike and scrape your knee, it feels sore, and if you're very tired your eyes may feel dry and gritty.

Touch is a sense we often don't think about, but where would we be without it?

Without our sense of touch, we wouldn't feel pain. We might rest our hands on a hot pan without noticing the burn. We might also be covered in cuts, scrapes and bruises. Because we would not feel the cold, we might go out in icy weather without warm clothes, and so become ill. What else might happen if we lost the sense of touch?

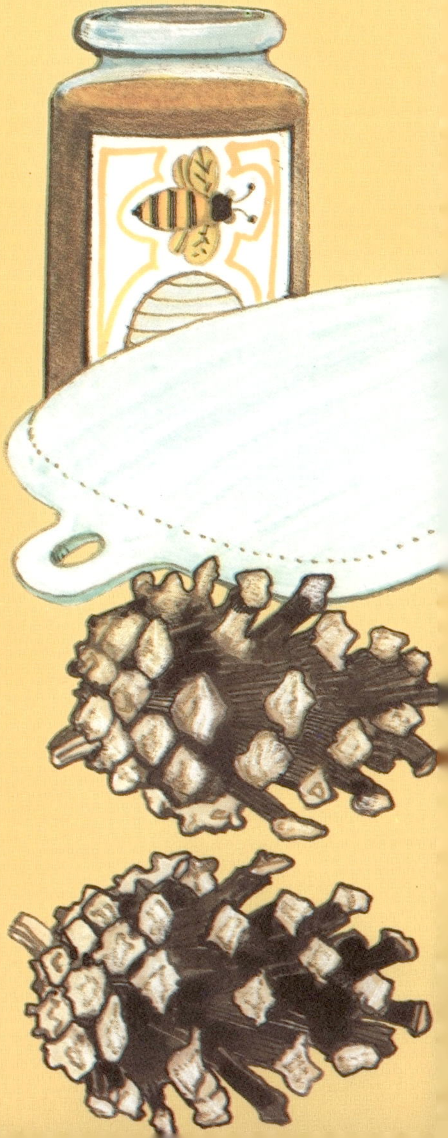

Touch can tell us many things. You could probably tell what each of these things is just by touching them.

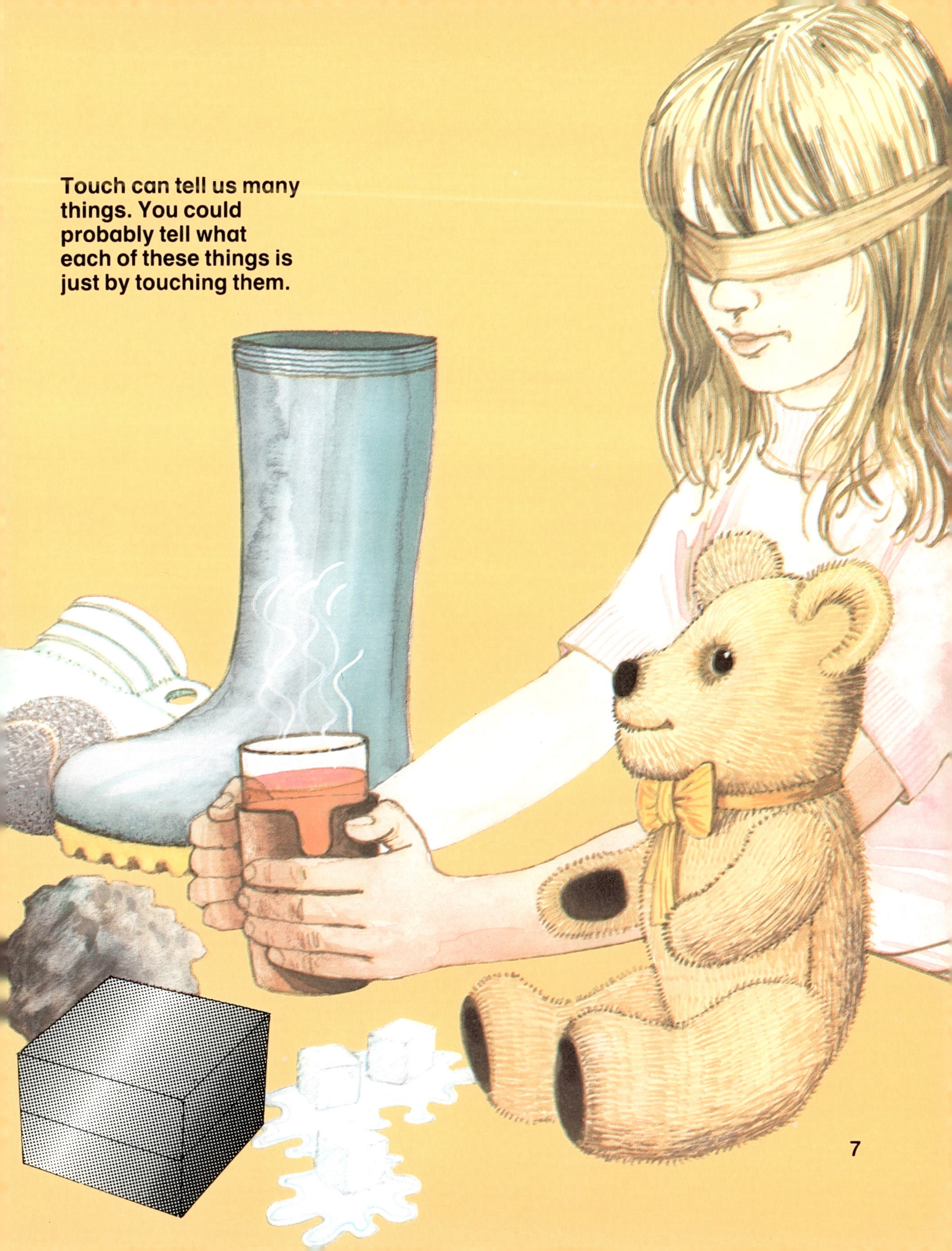

Sensitive and insensitive

A cat slips easily through narrow gaps. Its whiskers tell it if the space is wide enough for its body.

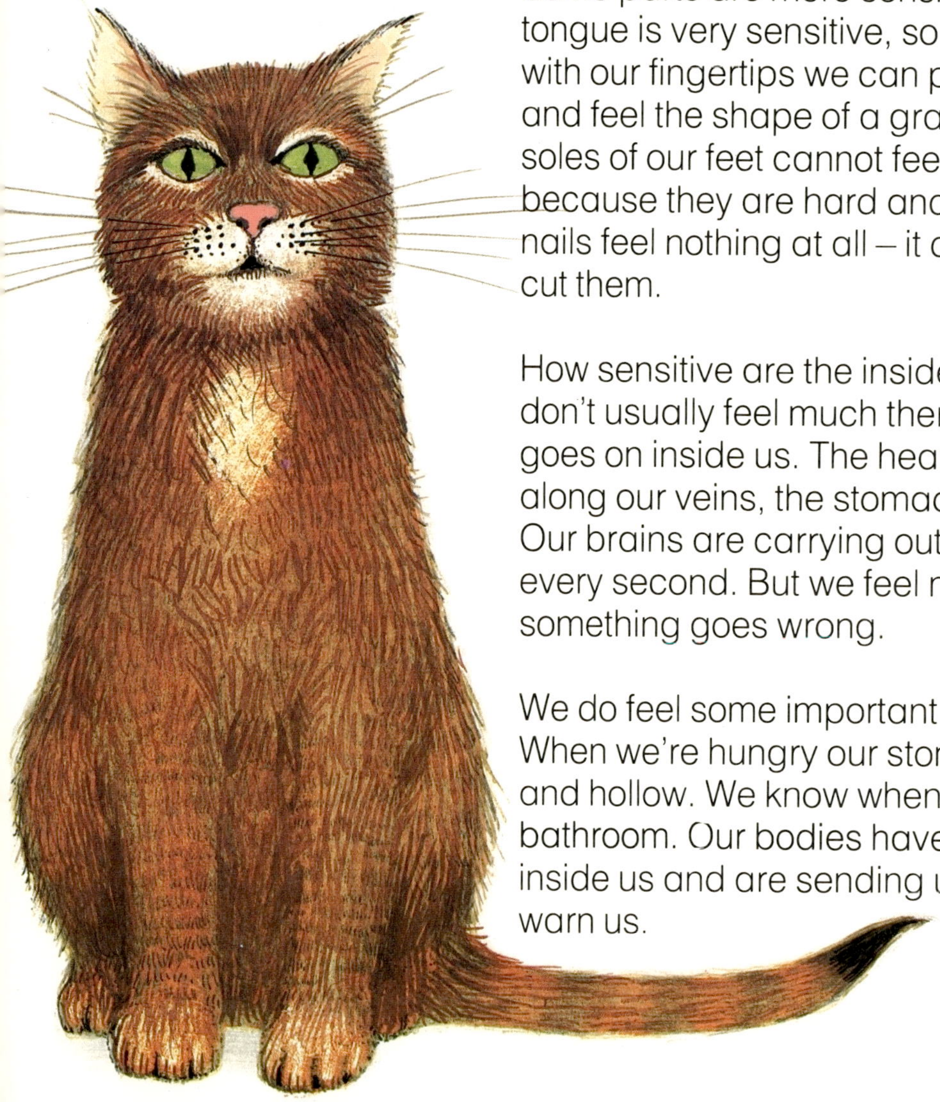

Things touch us all the time – our clothes against our skin, the air, and the ground under our feet. But we don't feel these things all the time, and not all parts of the body are equally sensitive to what touches us or what we touch.

Some parts are more sensitive than others. The tongue is very sensitive, so are our lips, and with our fingertips we can pick up tiny objects and feel the shape of a grain of rice. But the soles of our feet cannot feel things easily, because they are hard and insensitive. Hair and nails feel nothing at all – it doesn't hurt to cut them.

How sensitive are the insides of our bodies? We don't usually feel much there even though a lot goes on inside us. The heart is pumping blood along our veins, the stomach is digesting food. Our brains are carrying out many difficult tasks every second. But we feel none of this unless something goes wrong.

We do feel some important events inside us. When we're hungry our stomachs seem empty and hollow. We know when we need to go to the bathroom. Our bodies have sensed a change inside us and are sending us messages to warn us.

Touch is even more important to some animals than it is to us. Rabbits, cats and mice have whiskers which touch things. As they move through gardens or fields their whiskers brush against objects. In this way they tell whether a gap is wide enough for them to pass through.

Some snakes can tell how far away their prey is by sensing the heat of the other animal's body. A snail knows the world mainly through touch. Tap its "horns" and it will curl into its shell. Sea anemones have many tentacles, like a fringe, and these use touch to tell them that food is near.

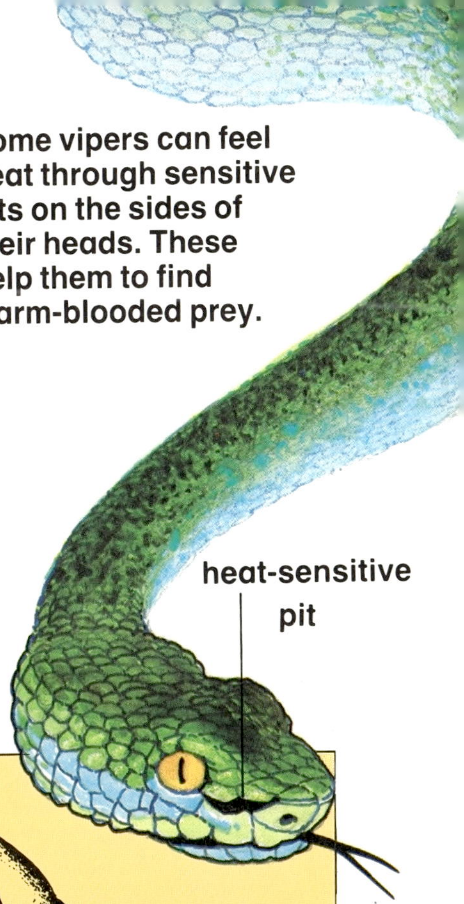

Some vipers can feel heat through sensitive pits on the sides of their heads. These help them to find warm-blooded prey.

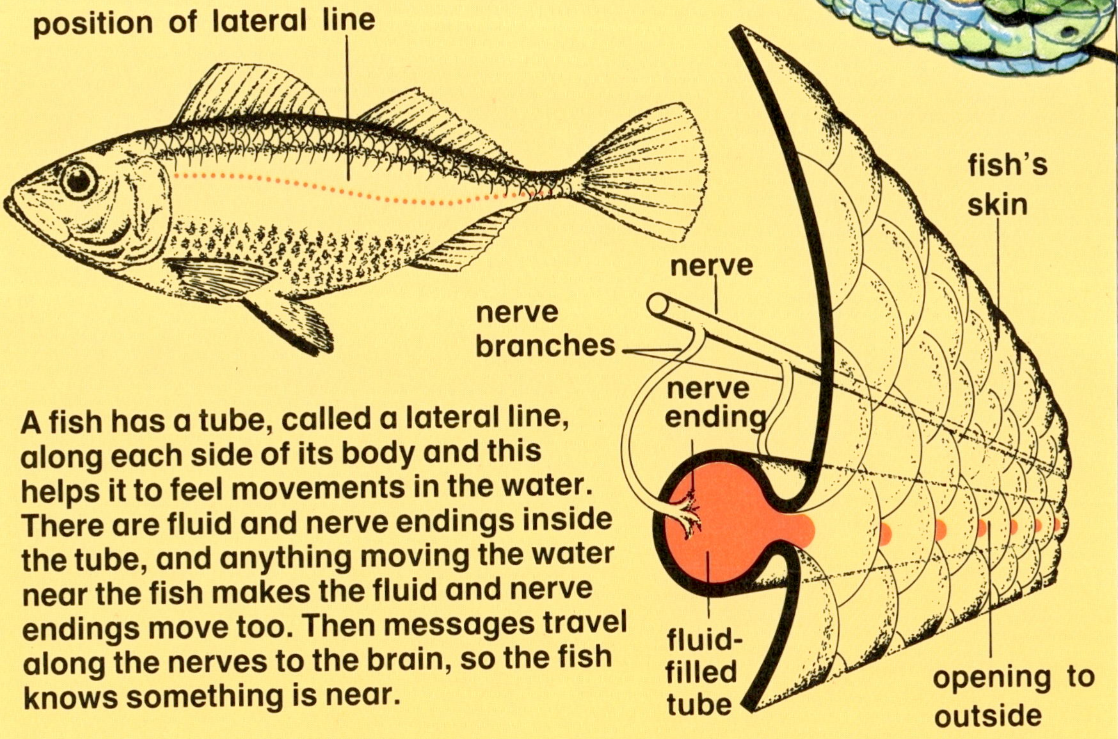

A fish has a tube, called a lateral line, along each side of its body and this helps it to feel movements in the water. There are fluid and nerve endings inside the tube, and anything moving the water near the fish makes the fluid and nerve endings move too. Then messages travel along the nerves to the brain, so the fish knows something is near.

HOW TOUCH WORKS

The skin

Skin protects us by keeping out dirt, germs and the Sun's rays. It helps in other ways too. It keeps moisture inside our bodies, and shields us against wetness from outside, because it is waterproof. It stretches when we move or flex our muscles because it is elastic.

Skin has two layers. The top layer, called the epidermis, is very thin and often flakes off as bits of dead skin. The second layer, the dermis, has blood vessels and nerves in it. It is these nerves which end in the skin that give us our sense of touch.

Human skin contains millions of nerves. These receive different sensations according to what we touch.

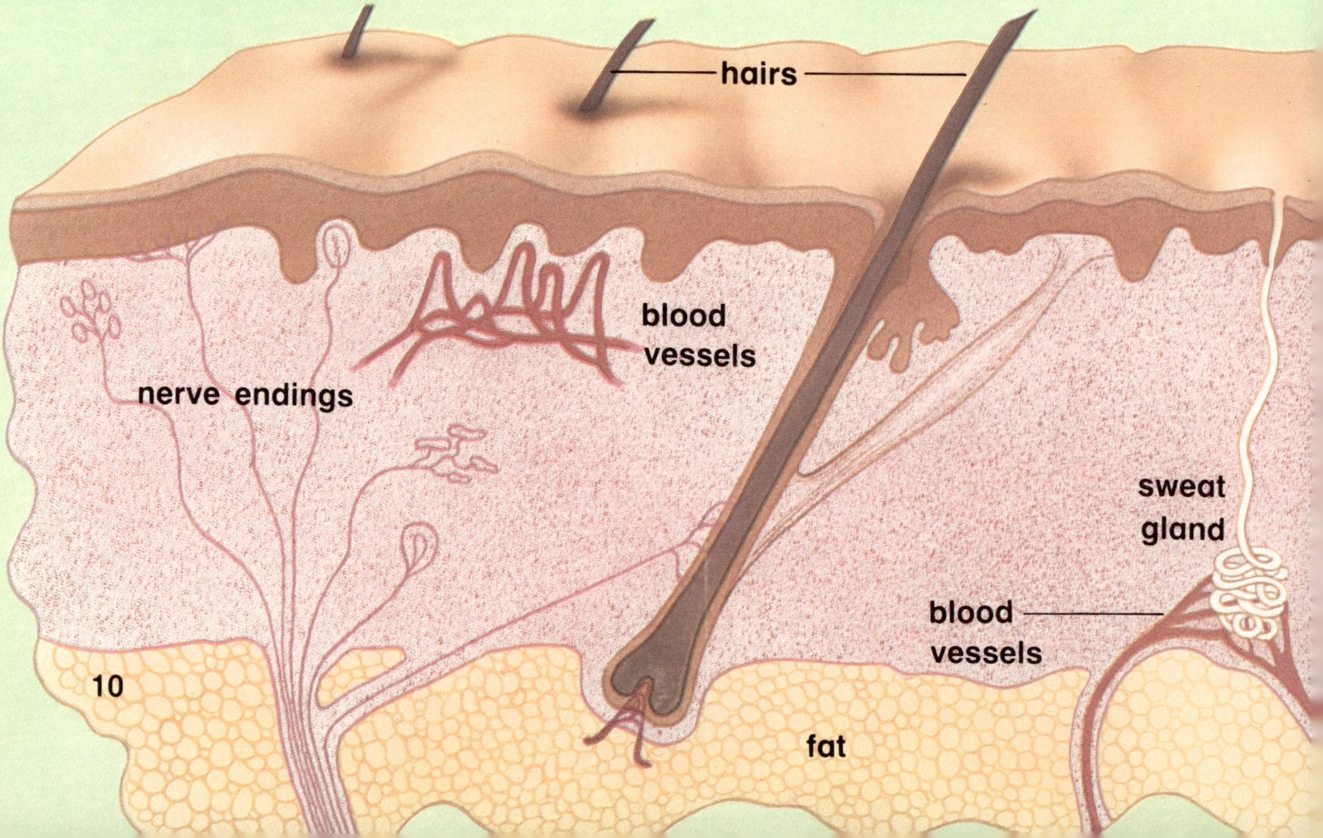

Your skin contains millions of nerve endings. Nerves are like tiny threads inside the skin which send messages to the brain about whatever we touch.

Nerve endings, or receptors, are like tiny switches or triggers which are set off by touch, pressure, heat, cold and pain. Some receptors are more sensitive to one type of sensation than to others. Hair and nails have no receptors and so feel nothing.

Skin receptors send messages in the form of electricity along chains of nerves to the spinal cord. This is made up of a large number of smaller nerves, and lies protected inside your backbone. Messages from the nerve endings run up the spinal cord to the brain. It may store the message or make the body react to it.

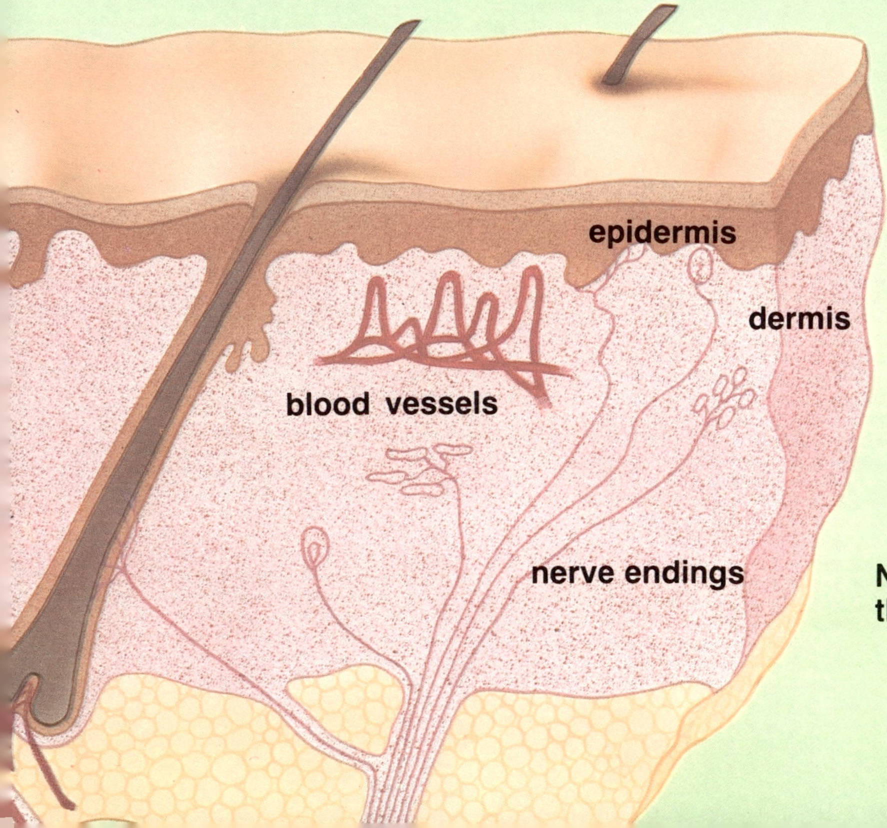

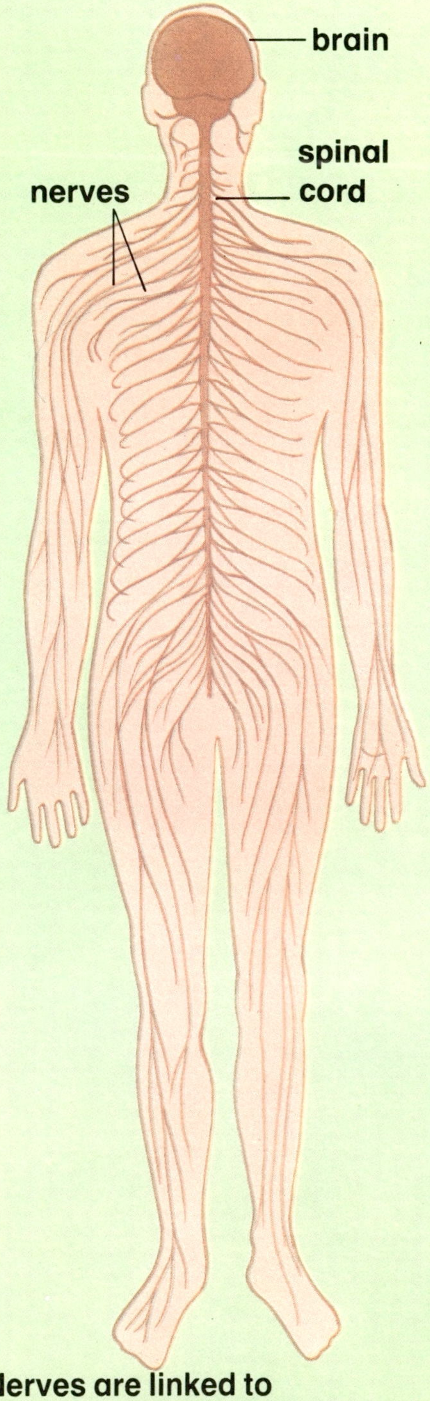

Nerves are linked to the spinal cord.

Reacting to touch

Here, the parts of the body with most feeling are shown biggest. They have more nerves so are more sensitive.

When we are awake, the brain receives messages all the time. It then sends orders to different parts of the body. Messages go back to the muscles through different sorts of nerves, called motor nerves. If we have touched something slimy or prickly, a message through the motor nerves tells us to snatch our hands away.

The parts of the body which have many nerves in the skin are most sensitive and need larger areas of the brain to deal with messages. These areas in the brain also store and remember some of the messages, so we know what to expect next time.

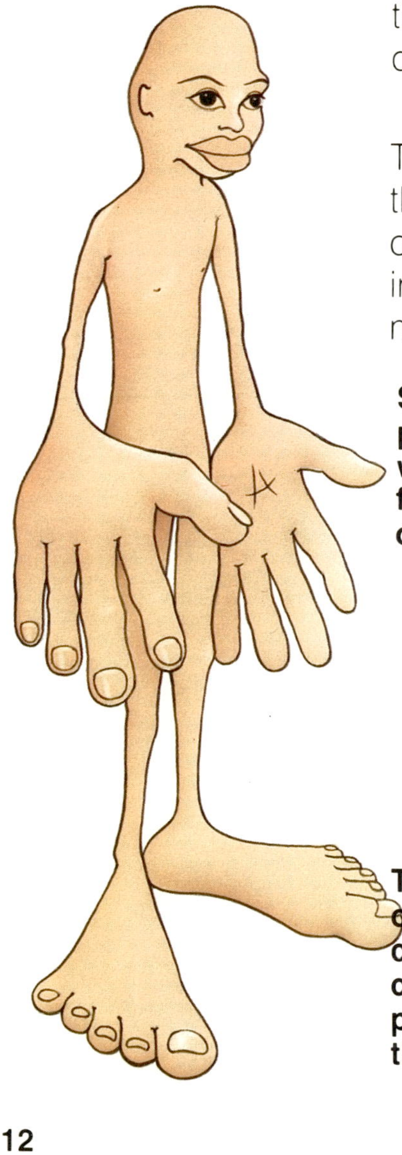

Sensory area – the part of the brain which feels sensations from different parts of the body.

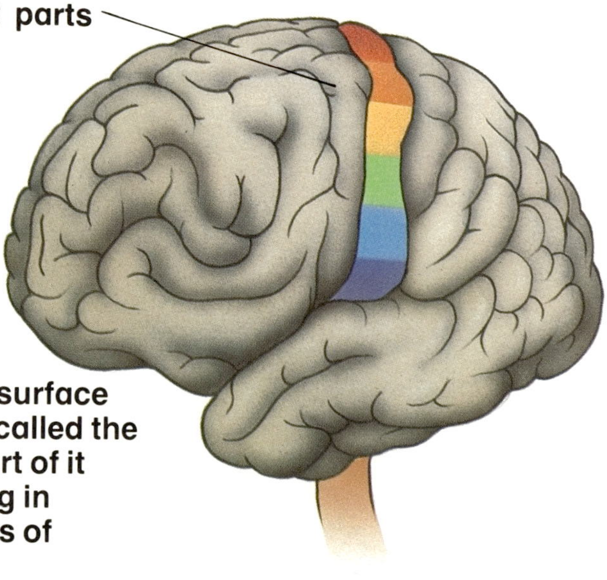

The crumpled surface of the brain is called the cortex. One part of it controls feeling in particular parts of the body.

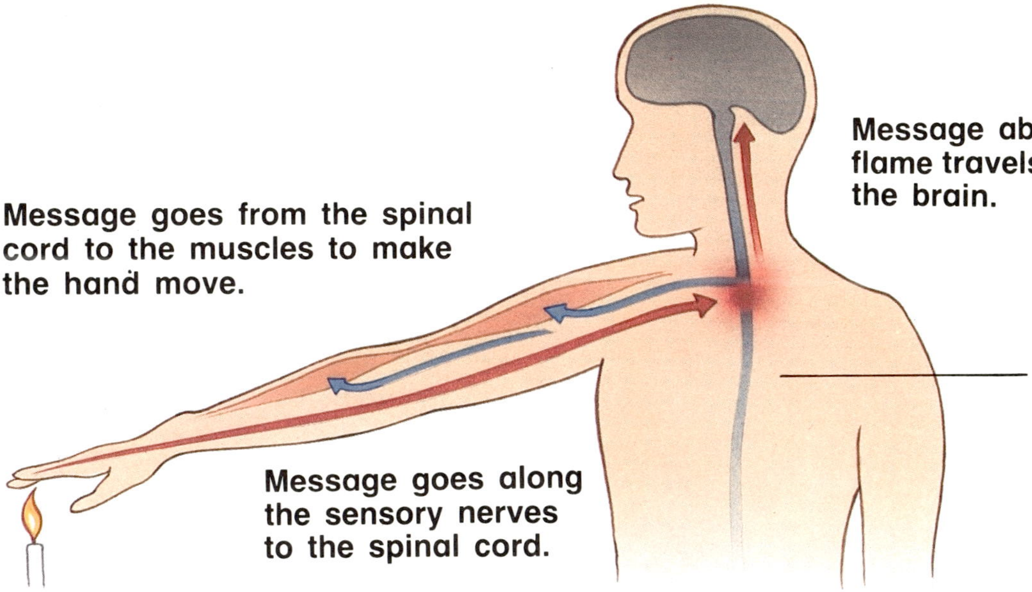

A flame burns the skin. Messages flash along nerves to the spinal cord. You pull your hand away before your brain knows what has happened. This is the spinal reflex.

The brain controls all our senses and actions. It is divided into different areas, each with a special job to do. Some parts control the workings of our organs, such as the heart and the lungs. Another part controls thought and memory. The largest part of the brain is the cortex, which forms a thick and folded layer around the upper surfaces and sides of the brain. A wide strip across the cortex deals with the sense of touch.

Sometimes we react before the brain knows anything has happened, and this is called a reflex action. This usually happens in an emergency. For example, if you grab a spool of thread without noticing a needle in it, you drop the spool and then cry out in pain. What has happened is that a message has gone straight from the sensory nerves to the spinal cord then out again along the motor nerves, before it ever reaches the brain. When the message does reach the brain you feel the pain, but you have already dropped the spool of thread.

Inside the body

Nerves in the skin help us to recognize the different objects we touch. But what happens inside us? A lot of important activities are going on out of sight there. The brain, heart, stomach, liver, and lungs are all working and so are other parts.

We feel only some of the things that go on inside the body. We can't feel food being digested. But if you have swallowed something too big, you feel it sticking in your throat.

We don't feel our brains working or blood moving in our veins. But we do sense certain things going on inside us. If you have eaten something poisonous, a message goes to the brain and you feel a pain in your stomach. And nerves in the bowel and bladder tell us when we need to go to the bathroom.

We feel something in our muscles too. Nerve endings there, called stretch receptors, tell us when our muscles are working hard. They tell us when they are tired too. This helps us know when to stop before a muscle is strained.

Nerves inside our muscles and tendons help us to know the position of our bodies. With our eyes closed we can reach out and touch nose, lips or chin. This is because nerves inside us send messages to the brain. The brain uses these messages to find out what the limbs are doing and where they are. So with our eyes closed, or in the dark, we can walk, sit, stand and reach out with our hands.

There are nerves in the bowel. They tell us when we need to go to the bathroom. If there is something wrong inside the bowel, the nerves make us feel a pain.

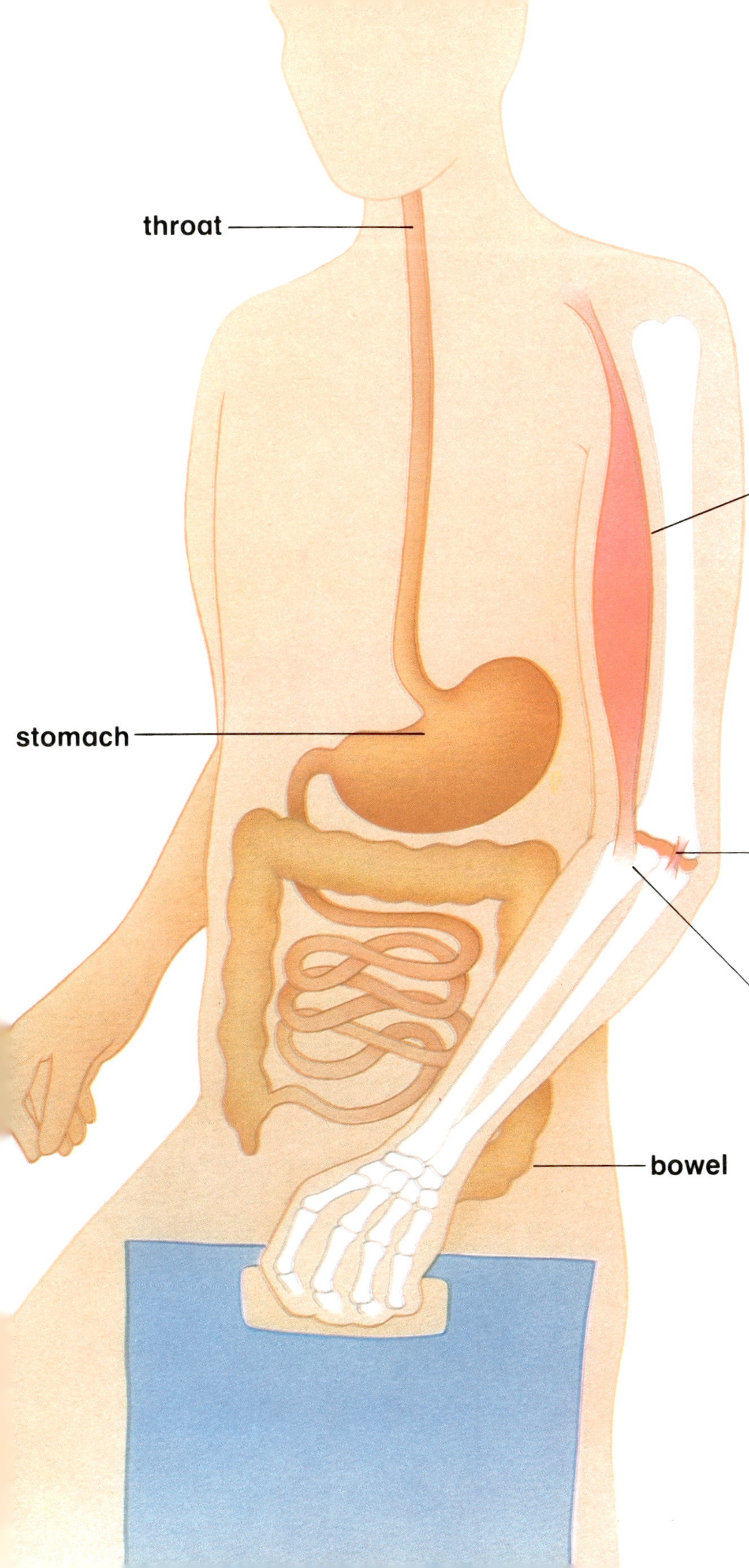

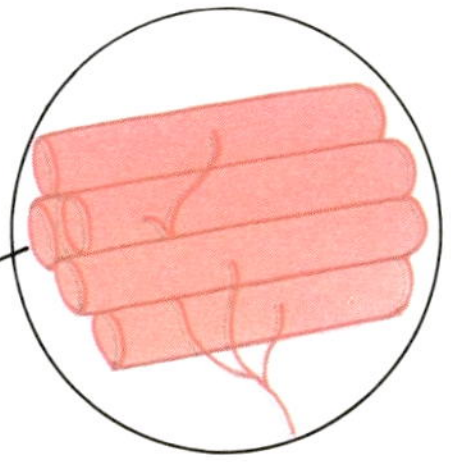

Nerve endings called stretch receptors lie inside muscles. They tell us how much the muscles are stretched.

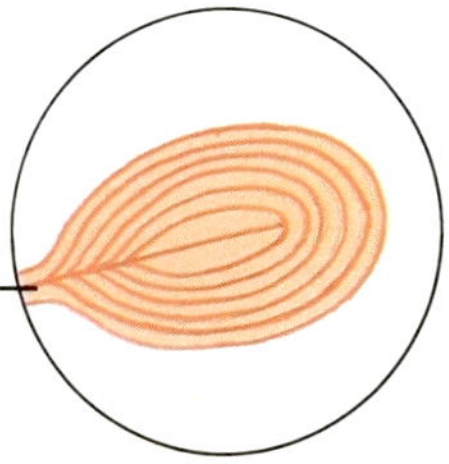

There are nerves inside joints, too. They warn us if the joint is under stress.

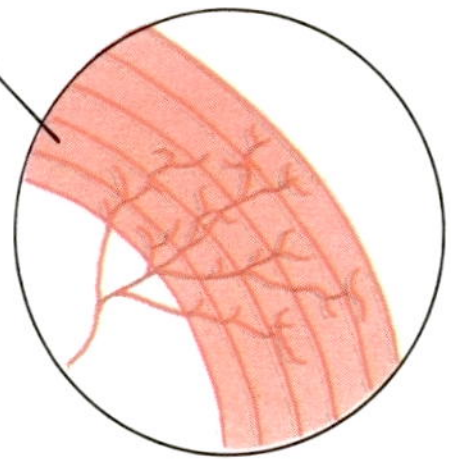

Stretch receptors in tendons measure strain there. Tendons fasten muscles to bones.

PRESSURE AND TOUCH

Exploring touch

If you run your finger over a table top you may feel tiny scratches or bumps. But if you do the same with your elbow, you won't feel the scratches or bumps. Why are some parts of our bodies more sensitive than others?

A part which is sensitive has more nerve endings clustered closer together. Some parts of the body are more sensitive to pain. Others are more sensitive to pressure or to temperature. What each part feels most depends on the type of nerve endings there.

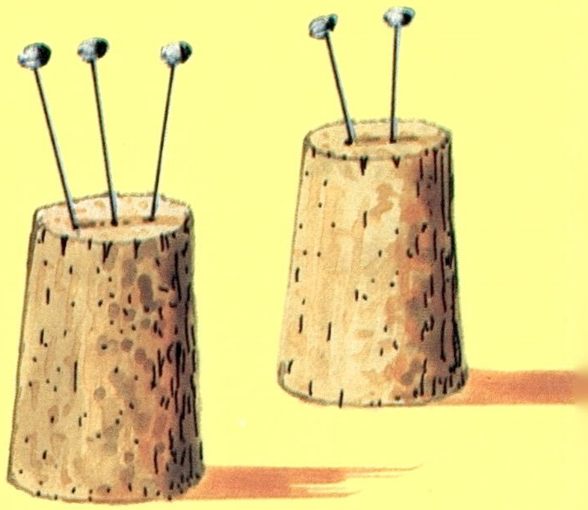

Use touch probes to help you explore the sense of touch. They are easy to make with corks and pins.

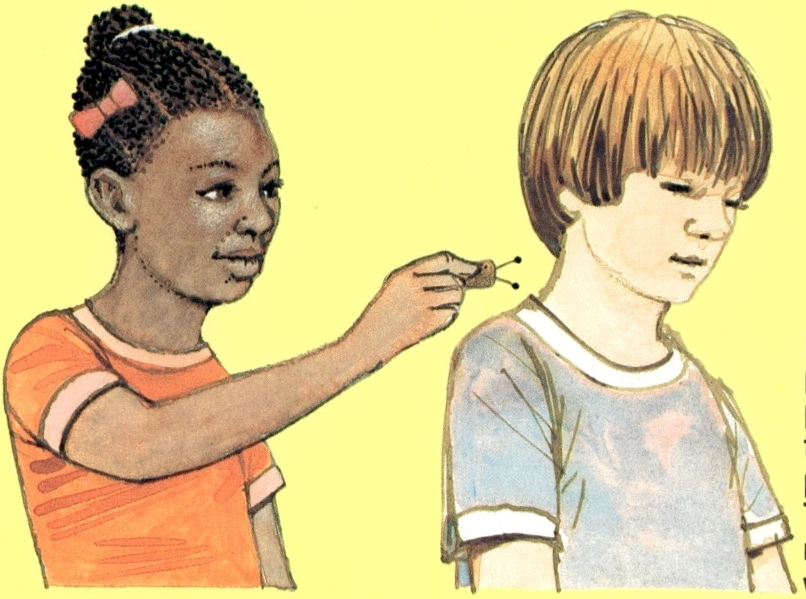

By touching different places with different probes you can find the more sensitive parts of the body. These have more nerves. Try it out with a friend.

Here are some experiments to help you explore the sense of touch with a friend. Get three corks and some pins. Stick one pin into the first cork, two into the second and three into the third. The pins must be the same distance apart in the second and third corks.

Use these corks as touch probes. While your friend keeps his eyes closed, gently touch his wrist with each probe. How many pins can he feel? Then test other parts of his body. Let him try it on you. Sometimes you will only feel one pin when there are two or three, depending on how sensitive to touch the skin is. Which parts of the body are the most sensitive?

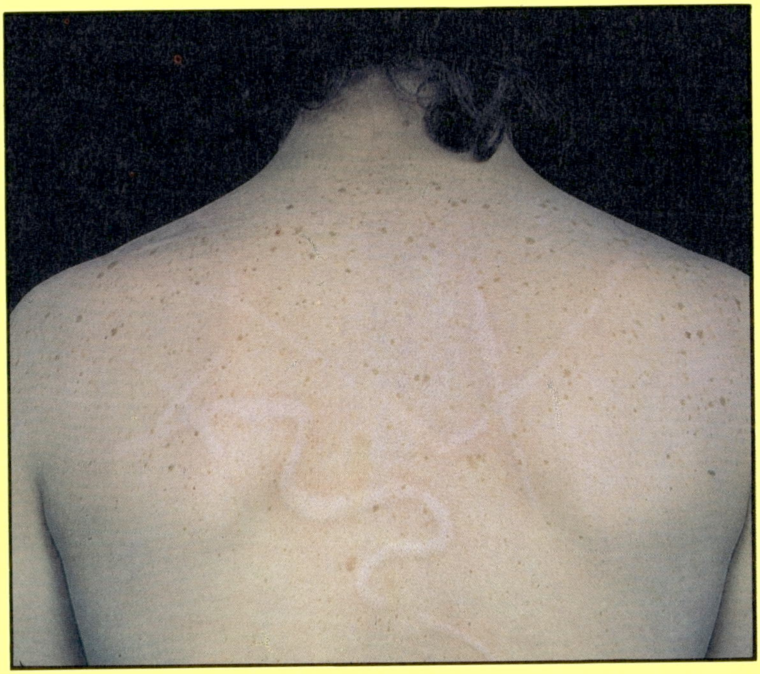

This person has the disease called Dermographia. His skin is so sensitive that it swells at even a light touch.

Ask a friend to put small objects in a box with a hole in the top. See if you can tell what they are by touch alone. Your brain remembers what things feel like and guesses what the objects might be. You won't always guess right!

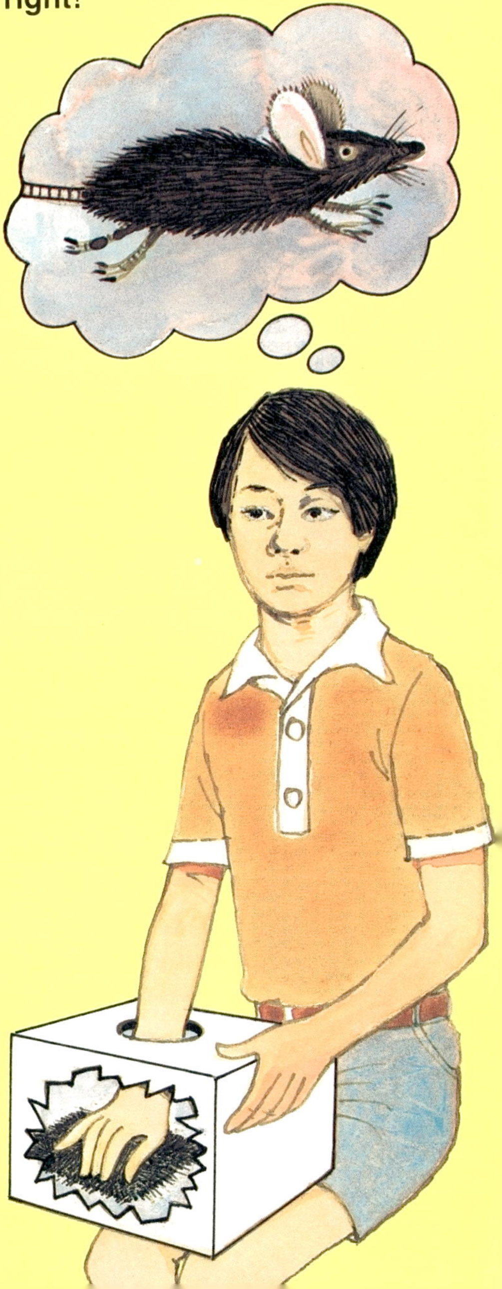

Using and losing touch

Touch is important for every movement we make. We feel our feet press on the pavement when we walk. And we know through touch when we lift our feet to step forward.

Could we walk without the sense of touch? Think about what it is like to have "pins and needles." You may sit in a way which keeps blood from flowing to your foot and stops messages from passing along nerves. We say the foot has "gone to sleep." You can't feel anything in your foot and can't move it. Then comes the tingling "pins and needles" feeling once the blood flows back into your foot.

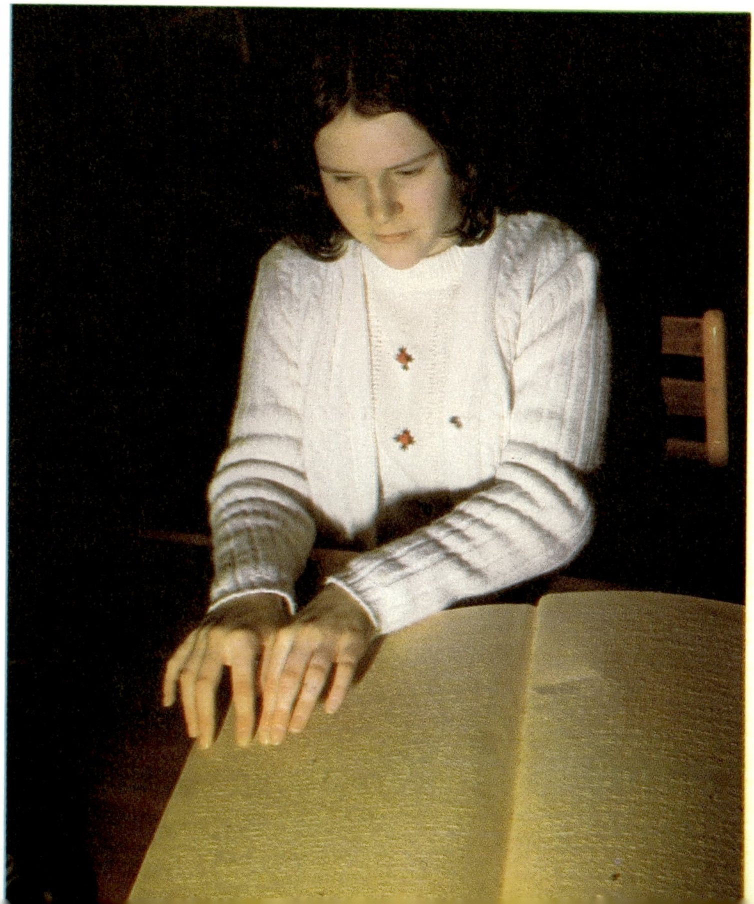

Blind people can read because of Braille. Raised dots on paper form words and sentences. You read Braille by touching the dots with your fingertips. Many books are printed in Braille.

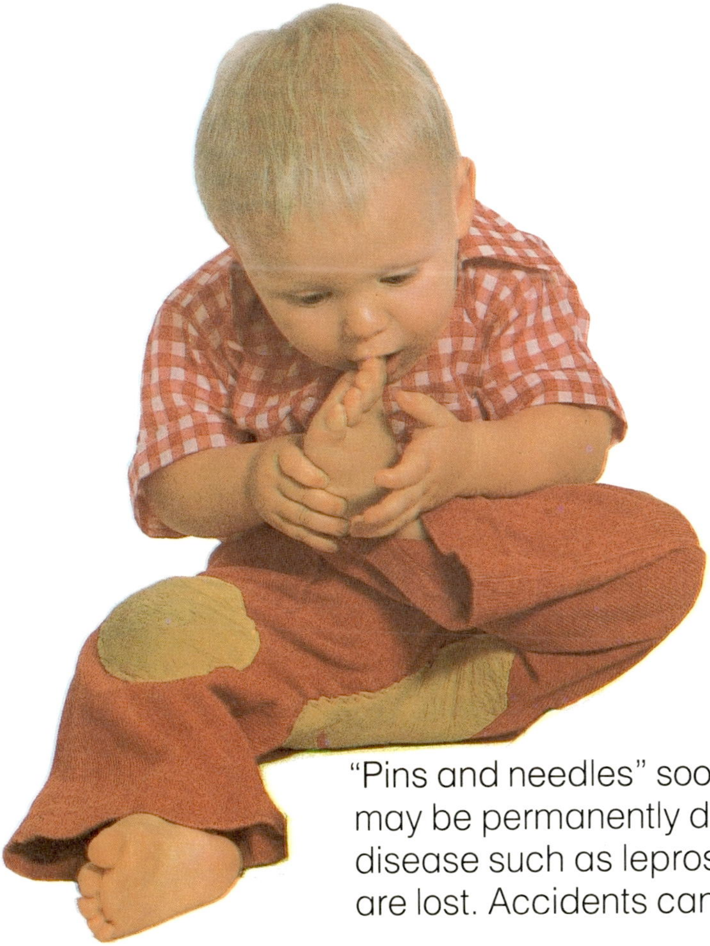

In the first months of life babies find out about objects by feeling them. They often feel things with their mouths. This could be dangerous so you should never give babies anything small enough to swallow.

"Pins and needles" soon goes away. But nerves may be permanently damaged through a disease such as leprosy. Feeling and movement are lost. Accidents can also damage nerves.

Someone who has lost part of a limb in an accident may sometimes feel as though the whole limb is still there. The parts of the nerves left still send messages to the brain although the nerve endings have gone. This is called phantom pain.

Some people rely on touch more than others. Babies put things in their mouths. This is a way of exploring the world. Blind people's other senses become very sharp to make up for the loss of sight and they may feel their way by touch. They can tell when they reach a street corner because they feel changes in air movements.

Exploring temperature

The same temperature may feel very cold to us one moment, but not so cold soon after. This happens at the beach. We grit our teeth before running into the ocean because we're afraid of the cold water, but a few minutes after plunging in, the water feels fine.

The same goes for heat. Let's say we swim in the adults' pool at the swim club. Then we get into the heated children's pool. At first it feels hot, but soon it's just warm.

This is because we react to changes in temperature rather than to the temperature itself. When we are used to a temperature we stop noticing it.

This experiment shows that we sense changes in temperature. One hand gets used to a bowl of warm water, the other to the feel of cold water. What would happen if you put both hands in another bowl of water between the two temperatures?

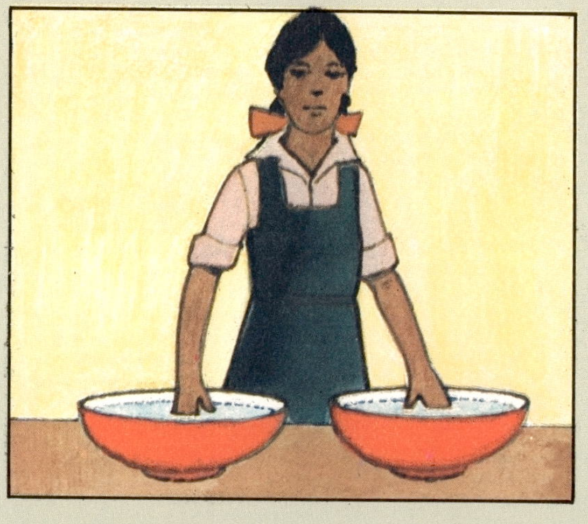

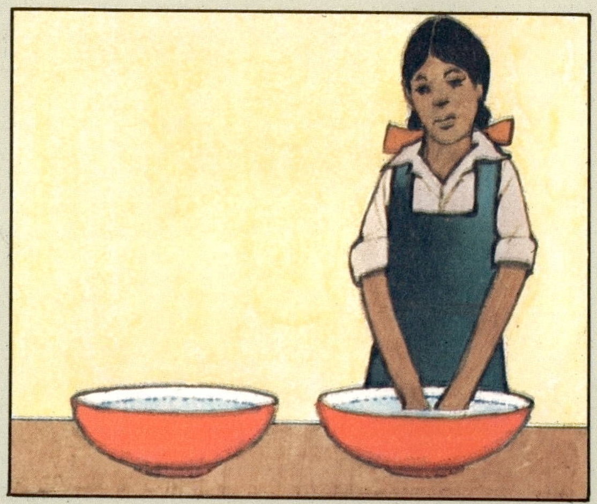

A baby's skin is very sensitive to heat and can be hurt easily. The water for its bath must be just the right temperature. People usually test the temperature with their elbows. The elbow is sensitive to heat because it has lots of heat receptors.

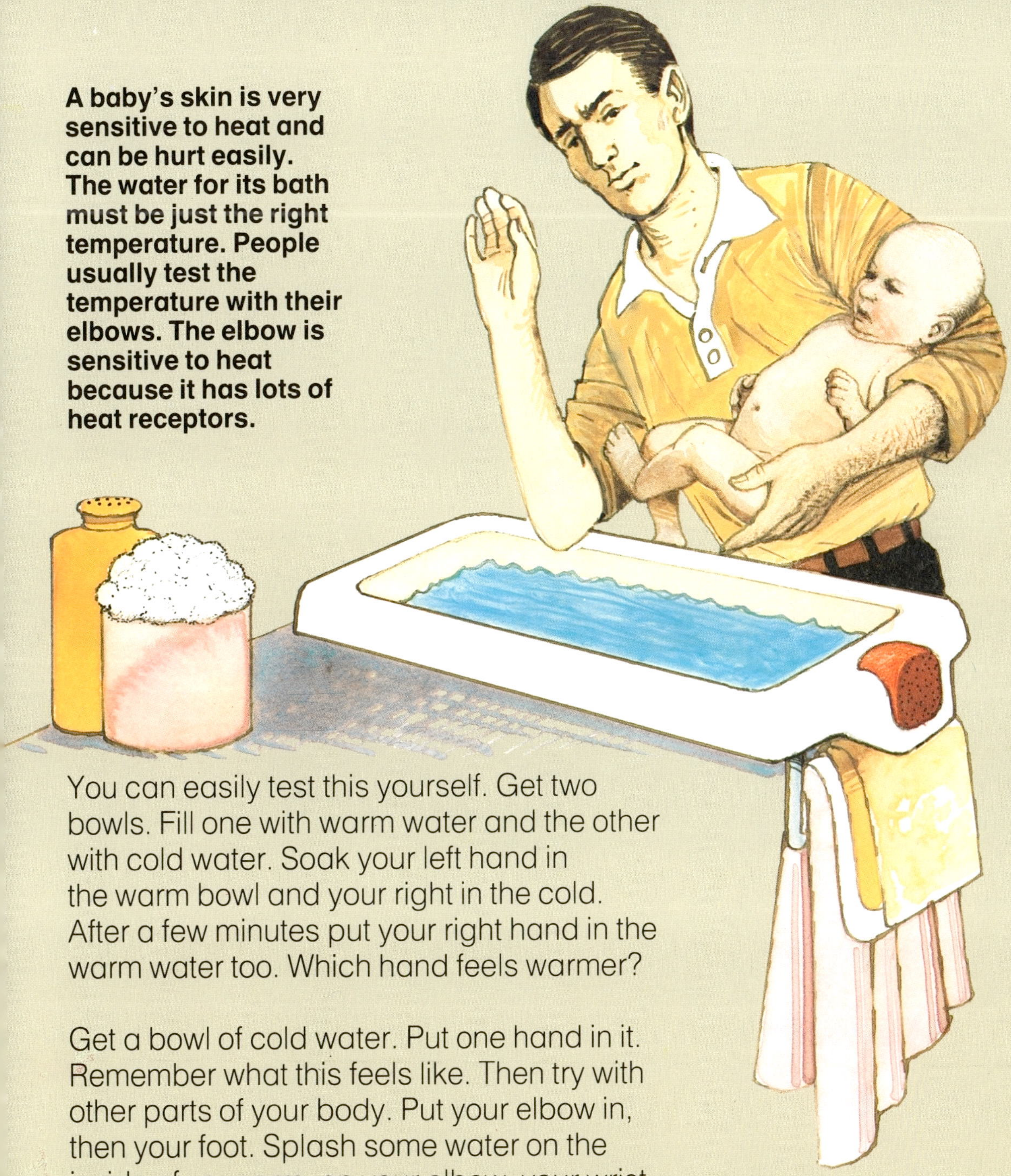

You can easily test this yourself. Get two bowls. Fill one with warm water and the other with cold water. Soak your left hand in the warm bowl and your right in the cold. After a few minutes put your right hand in the warm water too. Which hand feels warmer?

Get a bowl of cold water. Put one hand in it. Remember what this feels like. Then try with other parts of your body. Put your elbow in, then your foot. Splash some water on the inside of your arm, on your elbow, your wrist and on the back of your neck. Does the water feel as cold in each place? You can try this with warm water too.

Keeping cool and keeping warm

On a cold day we put on thick clothes to keep warm. But whatever we wear, the body always tries to keep its temperature much the same. If the temperature outside us falls, nerves tell the brain, and the blood vessels at the surface of the body quickly become narrower. Then less blood can reach the cool surface and so less heat escapes into the air.

But on a hot day we need to cool down. The more blood that flows through the skin, the more heat can escape to make us cooler. If you put one hand in a bowl of hot water, you will see your skin turn red as blood vessels near the surface become wider. Your body is increasing the blood flow in your skin so that you will lose heat.

Birds fluff their feathers in cold weather. The effect is like putting on a jacket. Air is trapped under the layer of feathers and keeps heat in.

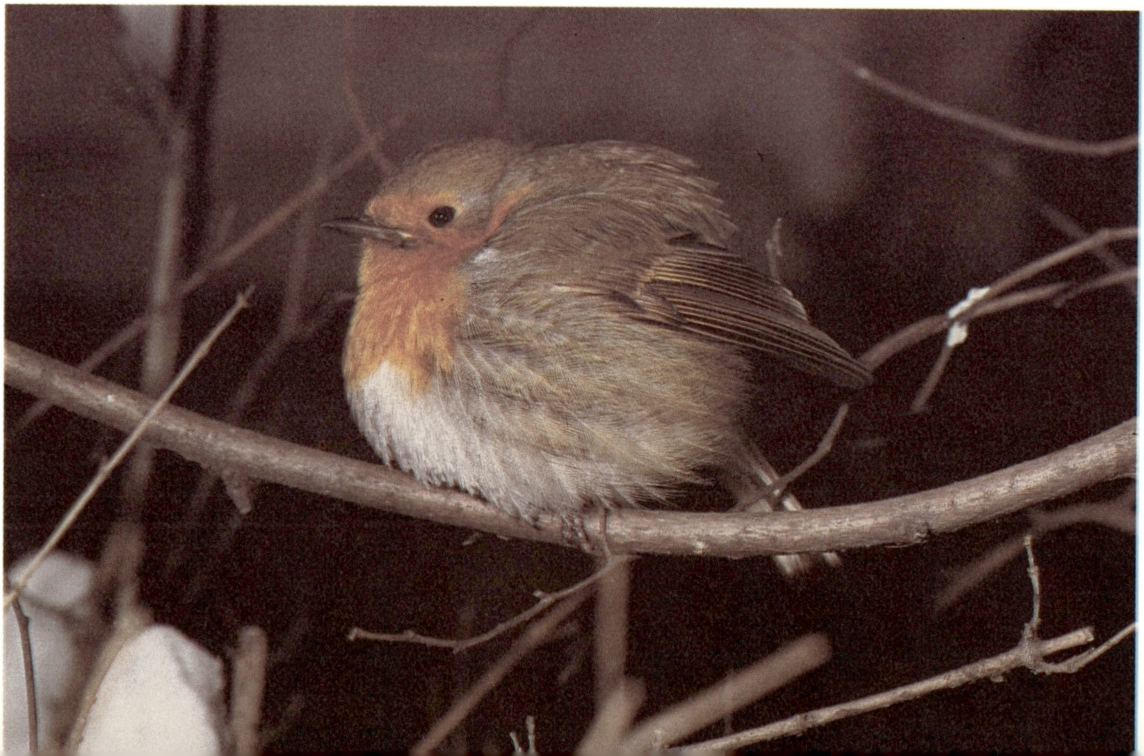

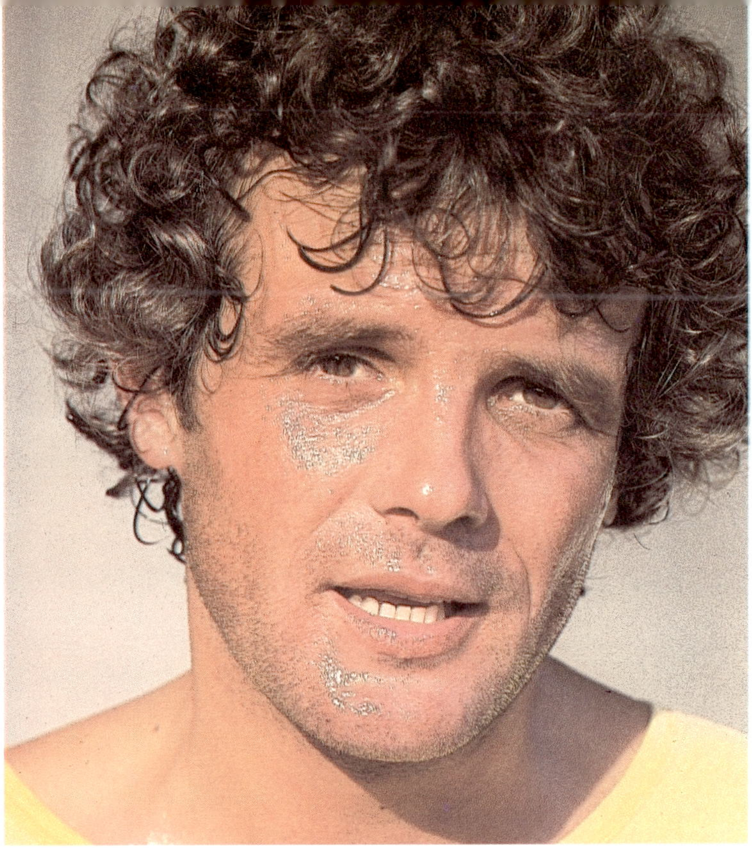

When we're hot, we sweat through the sweat glands in our skin. As the sweat on the skin dries, it cools us down. You can test this. Wet a finger and hold it in the air. Feel how your finger becomes cooler as the water dries.

Animals have many ways of keeping cool. A hippo wallows in cool mud or floats under the surface of a lake. But an elephant flaps its enormous ears. This helps cool the blood as it flows through the ears.

When a dog feels hot it pants so air cools its wet tongue. Blood passing through the tongue cools down too.

In cold weather birds fluff out their feathers. Air gets trapped in the feathers and helps keep heat in. Like birds' feathers, the hairs on our skin stand up to trap air when we feel cold. Tiny muscles move the hairs and show as "goose pimples."

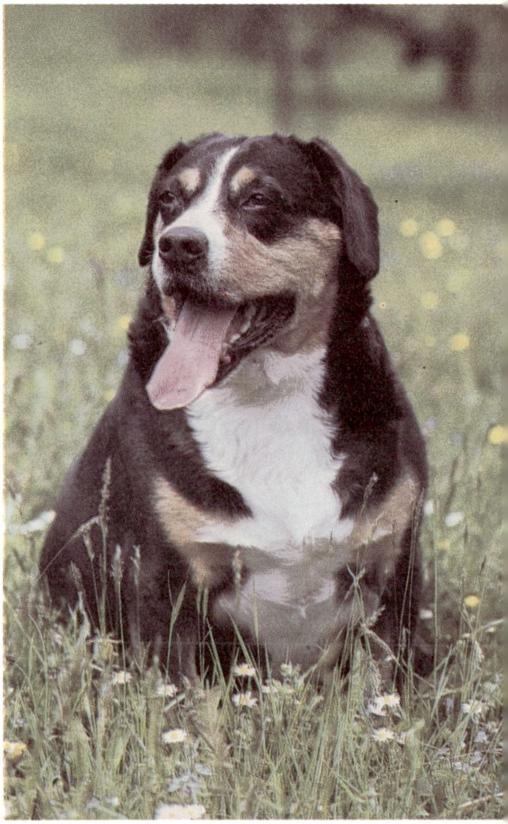

When a dog is hot it pants and hangs out its tongue. This helps it to cool down.

Too much heat or cold

Our normal body temperature is about 98.6°F. Small changes don't matter, but big ones do. Our bodies need to be at the right temperature to work properly. On freezing cold days signs around ponds warn us not to walk on the ice. Anyone who fell through would be soaked in freezing water. Soon they would not be able to feel or move and would die unless rescued.

If your body temperature falls, you lose the use of your muscles. If your body temperature drops to about 86°F, you lose consciousness. When the body reaches 77°F most people would die from the cold, but people have been known to recover after reaching 68°F.

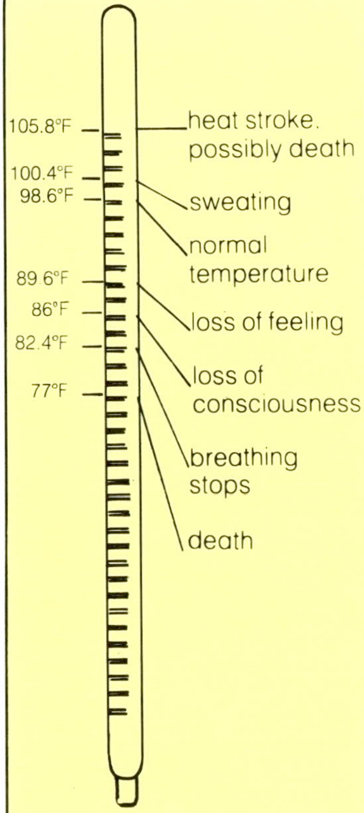

The temperature of the body may rise or fall. Small changes aren't dangerous. But this chart shows what happens when our temperature isn't kept close to normal.

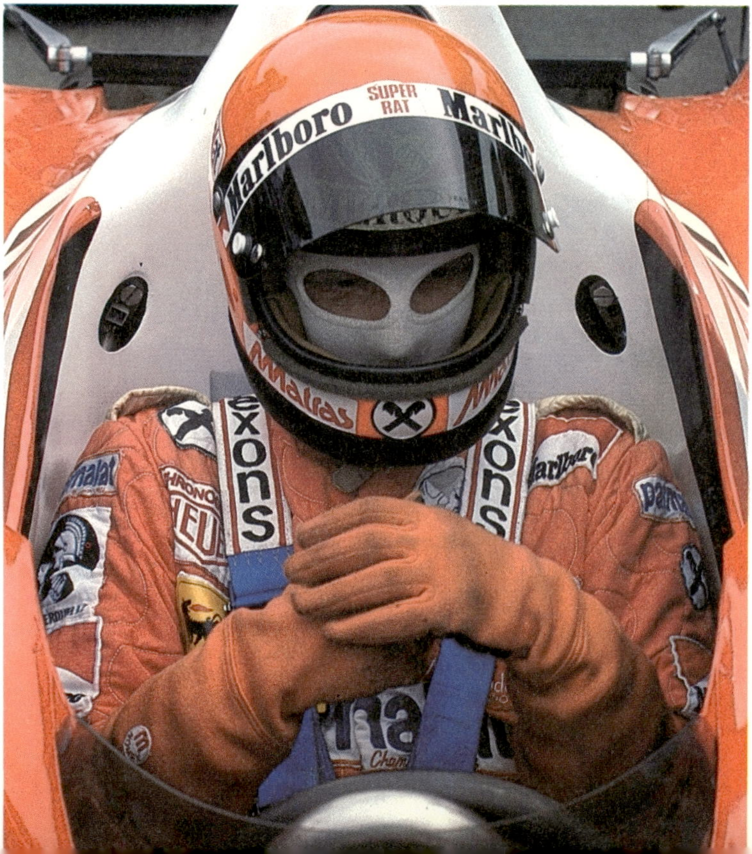

Skin is also damaged by too much heat. Racing drivers wear special suits to protect them in case the car crashes and then catches fire.

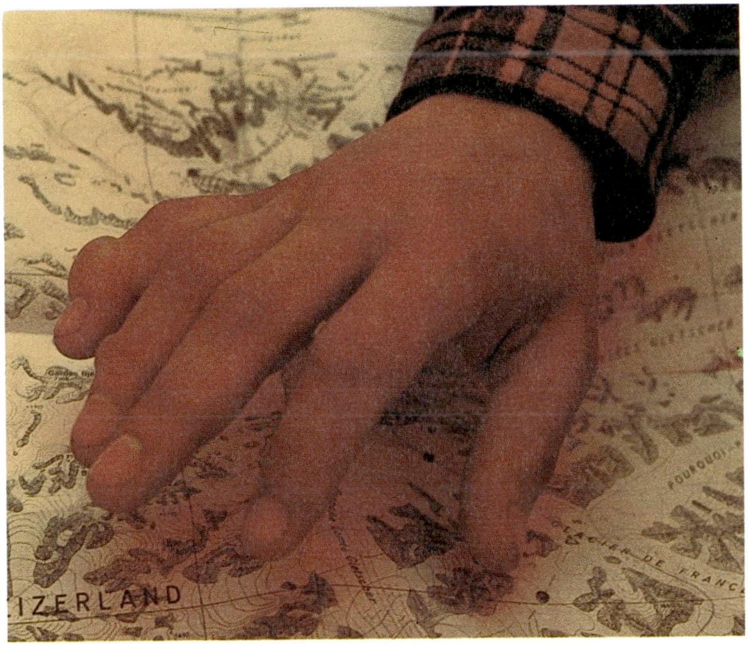

If we are very cold our blood cannot reach our fingers and toes because the blood vessels have narrowed so much. The skin becomes damaged and swollen, like a burn. This condition is frostbite. Frozen skin has to be warmed up gradually, because warming it too fast can cause even more damage.

An overheated body is in danger too. A disease may cause a rise in temperature, or the body can heat up when the temperature outside is very high, in a hot desert for example.
A rise in temperature makes the heart beat faster. As we sweat we lose salt, and this causes cramping in the muscles. If the salt is not replaced we may collapse. A body temperature of over 105.8°F can kill.

Intense heat damages the skin, causing burns which feel very painful. Small burns heal themselves but a large burn sometimes needs to be repaired with skin taken from another part of the body. This is called a skin graft.

FEELING PAIN

Itching, tickling or hurting

Pain nerves send messages to the brain when they are triggered. Other feelings like itching and tickling are also carried by these nerves, and by other nerve endings too.

Itching and tickling are like very mild feelings of pain. Tickling can even feel quite pleasant, but too much soon becomes uncomfortable. Itching is always unpleasant and a strong itch is very annoying.

Touch your skin with a piece of wool. What does it feel like? Try the feel of different objects. What hurts, what tickles, what makes you itch?

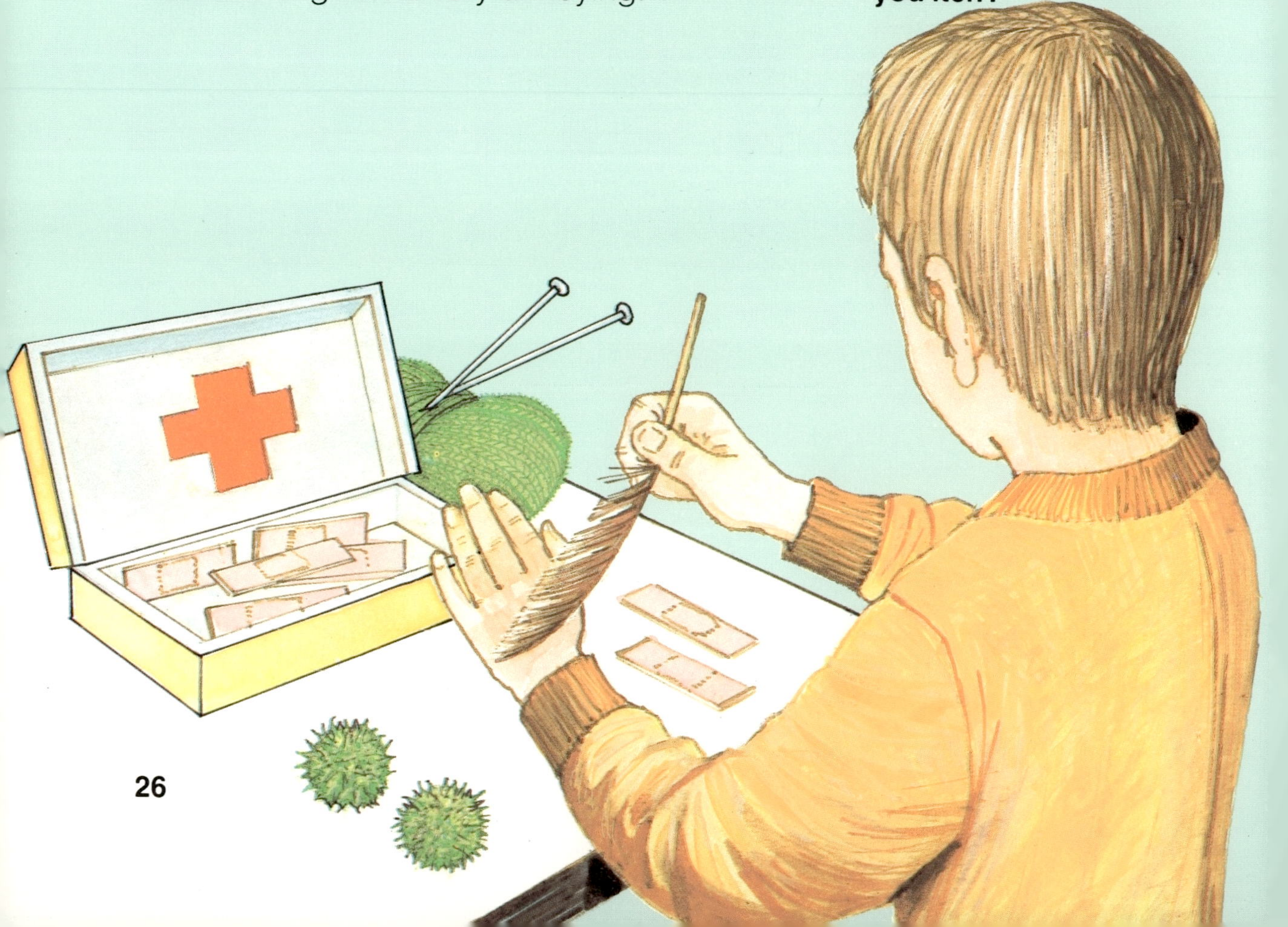

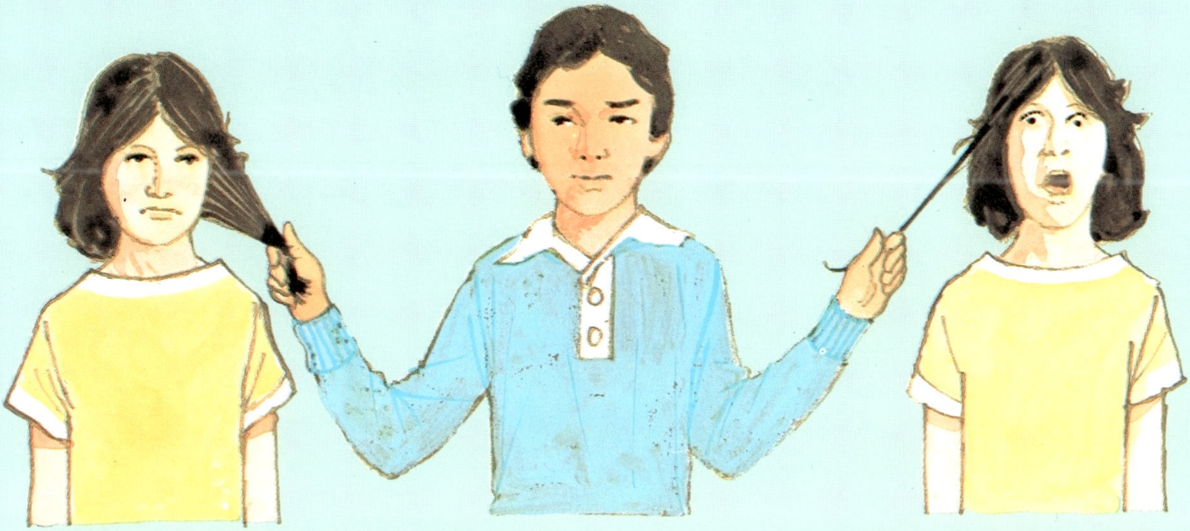

There are different types of pain. Some pain stings, another type might ache or throb. Pricking your finger with a pin hurts and so does having your hair pulled. But do they feel quite the same?

Having many hairs pulled hurts less than just a few because the pull is spread between all the hairs and so is not as hard on each one.

Pain is caused when receptors are triggered or damaged. Sometimes we start to feel better as soon as the cause of the pain is taken away. But if the nerves have been damaged they take time to mend and the pain may continue until they do.

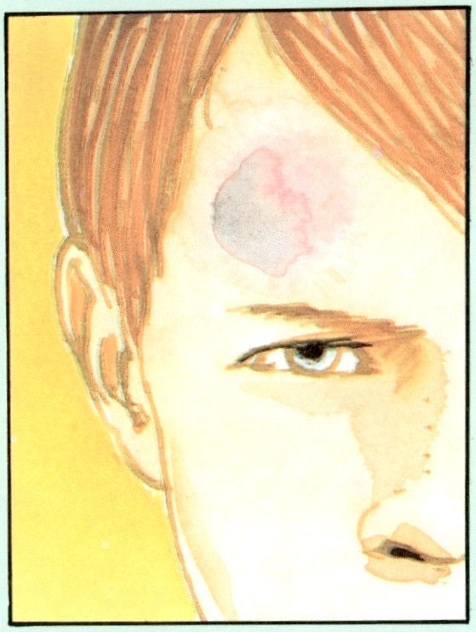

A bruise goes on hurting because blood vessels under the surface of the skin are broken and this affects nerve endings. As the bruise heals, the pain fades too.

We try to avoid pain. If we can't, we try to get rid of it quickly. But pain is also useful because it tells us something is wrong and makes us act quickly.

Broken blood vessels cause a bruise. Leaking fluid can collect and cause the skin to swell.

Painkillers

When we feel pain we act fast to get rid of the cause so we don't damage ourselves more. Pain makes us pull away from possible injury and it makes us go to the doctor for help. But pain is not only helpful, it also causes suffering and misery. People have always looked for ways of fighting pain.

It is easy to believe that the more seriously you are injured the more pain you feel, but this isn't so. Many important organs, including the brain itself, can be injured without pain. You only feel pain in an organ if it has nerve endings which are triggered by pain. Many organs inside the body have no pain receptors.

A needle stabbed into the skin is usually very painful. But healers trained in acupuncture can insert needles without causing pain. They believe that putting needles in the right places can make people healthy.

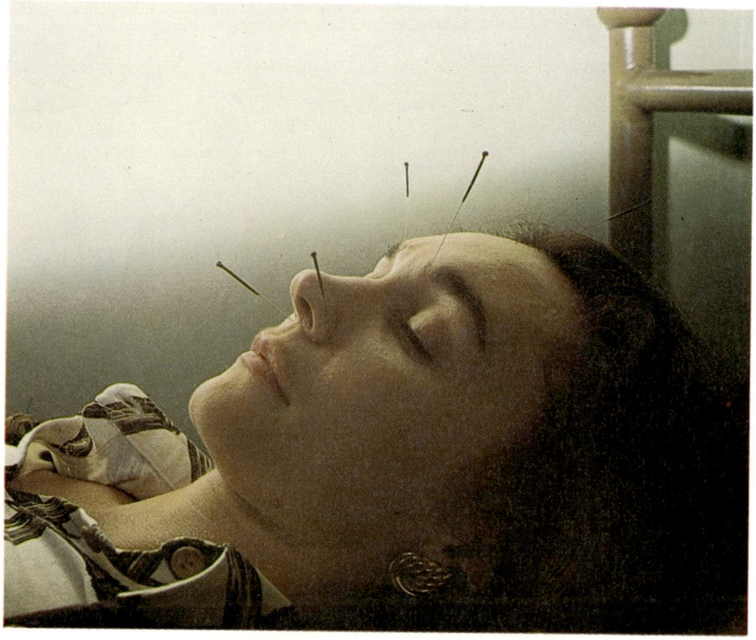

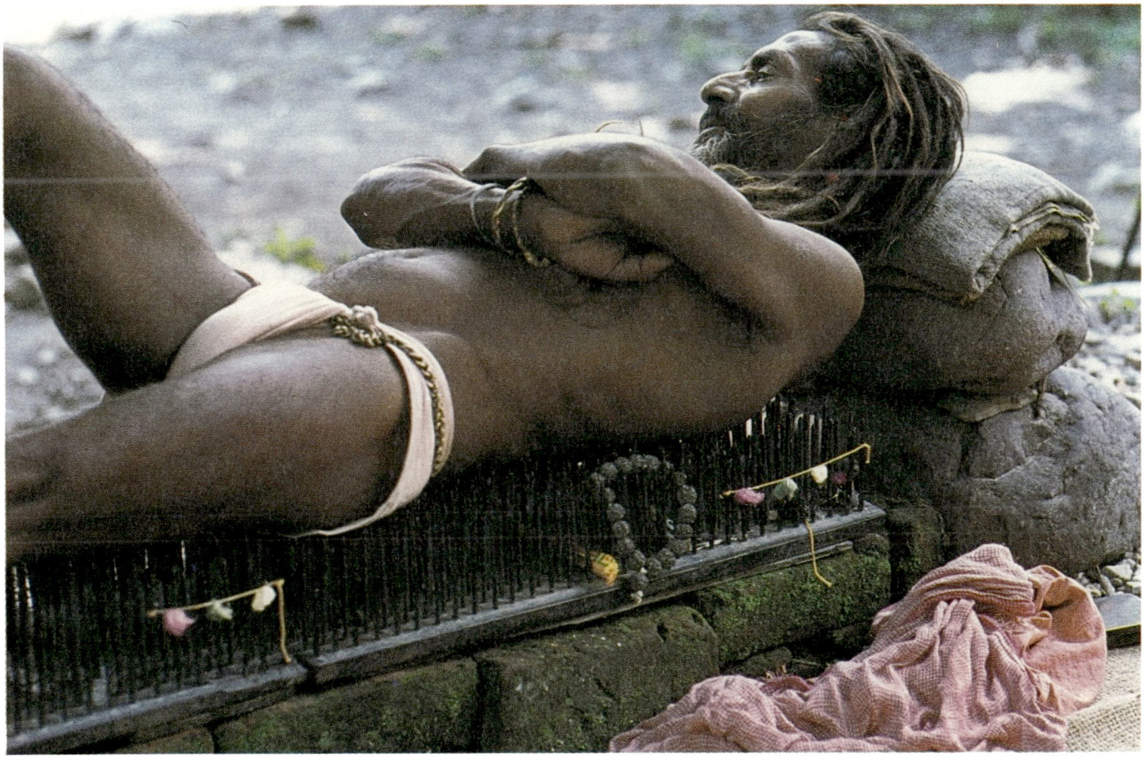

The mind has an effect on the amount of pain we feel. If we are relaxed we will feel less pain, but the more we are afraid of pain the more it hurts. Yogis in India believe the mind can control pain, and they have tried to train themselves not to feel it.

Does the mind control pain? Yogis believe it does. Some train themselves to feel no pain and can lie comfortably on a bed of nails.

Pain is usually controlled with drugs. They don't take away the cause but keep us from feeling the horrible sensation. Anaesthetics are used in operations. A local anaesthetic stops all feeling in a part of the body. A general anaesthetic acts on the whole body. Using anaesthetics, doctors can do operations without people trying to get away from the pain!

GLOSSARY, BOOKS TO READ

A glossary is a word list. This one explains unusual words that are used in this book.

Anaesthetics Drugs which take away feeling. Using these drugs, operations can be performed without pain.
Angina Pain caused by lack of oxygen in the heart. The pain may be felt in other parts of the body.
Cortex The deeply folded surface of the brain. One part of the cortex receives and sorts out messages sent by the nerves.
Dermographia A disease in which skin swells at the lightest touch.
Digestion The process by which food is broken down inside us so that it can be taken in and used by the body
Motor nerves Nerves which take messages from the brain to the muscles.
Muscles Bunches of fibers attached to bones. We can contract or relax our muscles. This makes the body move.
Nerves Threads or fibers which pass electrical messages to the brain from the sense organs and from the brain to the muscles. See also motor nerves and sensory nerves.
Paralysis Loss of movement in the body or a part of it. Paralysis is caused either by brain damage or damage to the motor nerves linking the muscles to the brain.
Phantom pain Sensation felt by someone who has lost a limb. The pain is felt as though the limb were still in place and hurting.
Receptor A nerve ending which reacts to different types of touch and sends messages along nerves to the brain.
Sensation A feeling caused when messages from nerve endings in the body reach the brain.
Sensory nerves Nerves which carry messages to the brain from the sense organs – ears, eyes, nose, taste buds and the nerve endings in the body which react to different touch sensations.
Spinal cord A collection of nerves inside the spine and linked to the brain.
Spinal reflex Quick reaction to something. The reaction is not triggered by the brain. Instead the link between the message and the reaction occurs in the spinal cord.
Tendon Strings of fiber that fasten muscles to bones.
Touch The sensations set up when receptors are triggered.
Yogi A person who practices yoga. a system of mental and physical exercises which was developed in India centuries ago.

BOOKS TO READ

Touch by Ed Catherall, Silver Burdett, 1982.
Touch Will Tell by Marcia Brown, Franklin Watts, 1979.
Touch, Taste and Smell by Brian Ward, Franklin Watts, 1982.
Looking at the Senses by Nina Sully, David and Charles, 1982.

INDEX

The **dark** numbers tell you where you will find a picture of the subject

1 2 3 4 5 6 7 8 9 10—JDL—95 94 93 92 91 90 89 88 87 86